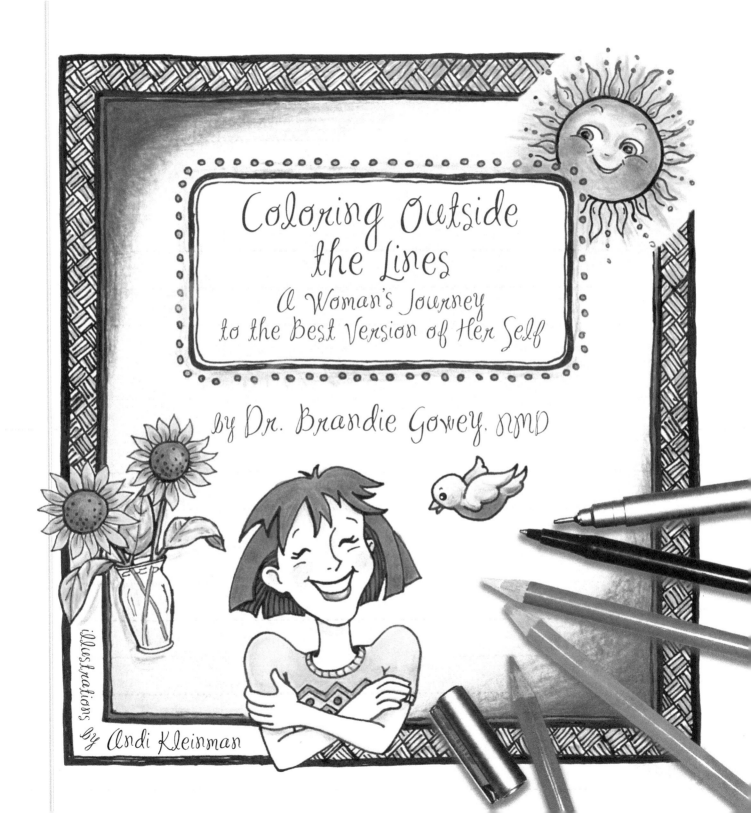

Coloring Outside the Lines
A Woman's Journey to the Best Version of Her Self

by Dr. Brandie Gowey, NMD

illustrations by Andi Kleinman

Coloring Outside the Lines
A Woman's Journey to the Best Version of Her Self

Illustrations by Andi Kleinman

Edited by Charoltte Fox

Published by
DR. DNA Press
Flagstaff, AZ

Printed in the United States of America

ISBN 978-0-9861850-2-1

Cover and Book Design by
Andi Kleinman

Proceeds from the sale of this book benefit medical research at DR. DNA Clinic. Learn more at *goweyresearchgroup.com*.

This book is not intended as a substitute for the medical advice of physicians and/or healthcare practitioners. In matters relating to their health, readers should regularly consult a physician and/or healthcare practitioner, and particularly with respect to any symptoms that may require diagnosis or medical attention.

Although the author and publisher have made every effort to ensure that the information in this book is correct at press time, the author and publisher do not assume and hereby disclaim any liability to any party for any loss, damage, or disruption caused by errors or omissions, whether such errors or omissions result from negligence, accident, or any other cause.

Create your life —
or life will create you.

Dr. Gowey, NMD

What is really hard, and really amazing,
is giving up on being perfect
and beginning the work
of becoming yourself.

Anna Quindlen

Please finish and color
the borders and illustrations
in this book.

Doodle on every page!

Enjoy being in touch
with your Creative Self!

Table of Contents

Table of Contents

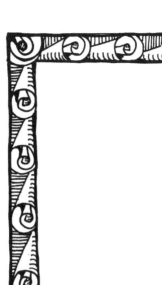

Introduction

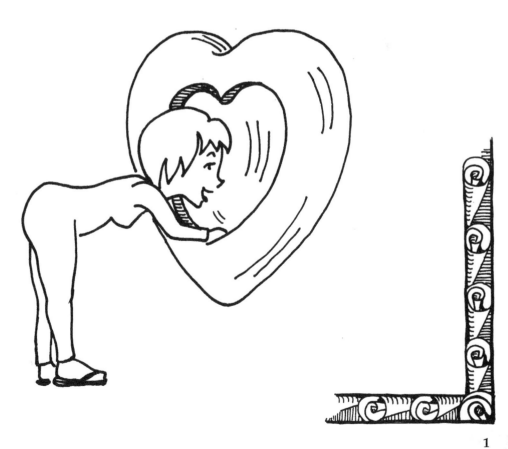

Introduction

New Year's Eve Day. I park my truck at the end of a nine-mile trail system that I hiked parts of before, but have never done end-to-end. I decided to make this New Year's Day special by challenging myself to hiking through this Valley, knowing I would most likely trek through deep snow.

I misjudged the depth of the snow, for within one mile I hit ankle-deep, then knee-deep, then calf-deep snow. My dog looked at me pleadingly to stop and go back to the truck, for her little legs were struggling to get through the deep snow. But I encouraged her, and as I did so I set my mind to keep going, even though my body was quickly becoming exhausted.

Hours later, we made it to the end of the Valley! I had traversed a very difficult and cold trail system, with no other companionship than my own thoughts and my dog. I encountered no other living soul until I reached the end of the trail.

Logic would say to never do this hike in the middle of the winter, alone, through deep snow. My heart and soul, however, had something else to say. Desire to experience life and to feel that a challenge was overcome, made me feel as though I had really been living!

How many of us play it safe? Or wait for a partner to tell us we can do something? Or let fear get in the way of doing something until we have a partner? How many of us are not willing to spend time alone?

This journal is my way of helping you search your heart to work out the answers to questions such as these. Playing it safe stops us from living.

So open your heart and mind, gather your pens and pencils, crayons and markers and don't be afraid to

Color Outside the Lines!

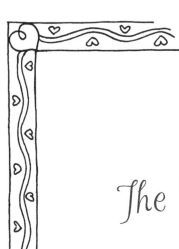

The Power of Loving Yourself

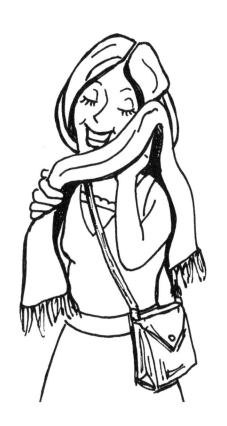

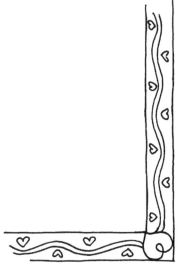

The Power of Loving Yourself

There is something about a woman's heart and spirit that desires a connection to a partner. We feel a yearning for love, affection, romance, and appreciation. We want that partner who will stand by our side, be good to us, take care of us, see to our needs, be loving, affectionate, help us meet our goals, or help us raise our children. We want the Cinderella fairytale. We want to be seen as beautiful!

The craving for this attention and affection drives us to distraction. We will go to no end to make ourselves beautiful and appealing to a potential mate. This is especially true when we are single. This craving in our heart is the focus of many a conversation over a cup of coffee, as well as hours and hours of situational analysis with friends, wondering, "does he/does she like me?"

However, the longer I live and the more I connect to my inner self and follow my joy, the more I realize that the desires we feel is actually a craving for ourselves.

Coloring Outside the Lines: I love myself.

Isn't it fun to pick out a new outfit? I would like you to plan out an afternoon or night to yourself. Go to your favorite clothing shop and pick out ANYTHING YOU WANT! You get just one item. Allow yourself to slowly go over the clothing options at this favorite store, try on a number of items, and pick out just one absolutely amazing outfit!

Then go home and get spiffed up, and take yourself out to dinner in that special outfit. How does it feel to be good to yourself?

Putting Yourself First

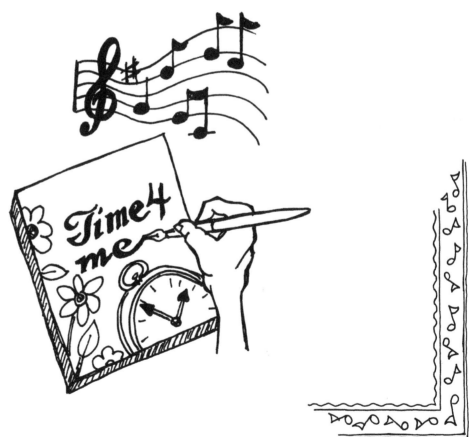

Putting Yourself First

One of the most important things you can do is take care of yourself. If you keep yourself healthy and happy, you can care for others. If we take care of others at the expense of ourselves, we get tired. And if we get tired, we get impatient. And if we get impatient we do things we wish we hadn't, like yell at those closest to us. And once we do that, we start to strike out, or give up, or quit whatever task we were doing.

Don't ignore your heart! Take time for friends or anything that builds you up. Build self-care into your lifestyle and you will be amazed at how much better you can take care of your work, friends, and family. Taking care of yourself really is the most important thing, and in reality, the most unselfish. It gives you the grace to move through your life and actually enjoy it!

Coloring Outside the Lines: I put myself first.

There are simple ways you can make sure to take good care of yourself. I have an hour I reserve every night for just me: I brew up a nice cup of tea and slink away to my art room, where I listen to classical music and either write (this is where I wrote this journal!) or do some illustrations for my mom's books. I LOVE this time. I savor it and I almost can't wait for it!

Think about what you want to do for putting yourself first. It doesn't have to be a difficult process. Pick something simple you can incorporate into your everyday routine. What do you love to do that gives you the time you need for yourself?

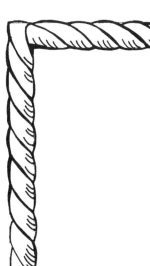

Women are Incredible

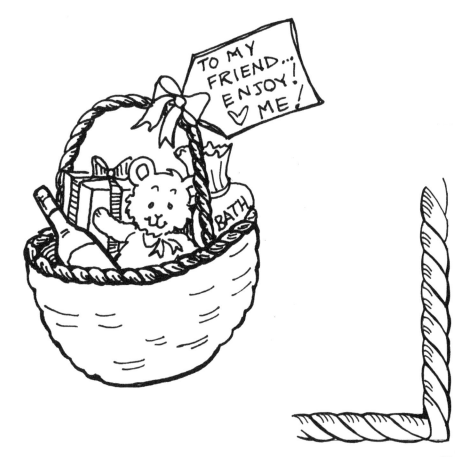

Women Are Incredible

Our capacity to love and give is amazing! Here is an example:

I have a friend with two adult children addicted to drugs. Both of her sons have been in and out of jail, work, and relationships. One of her sons is living with her. The other has had two children with a Methadone-addicted girlfriend. Both her grandchildren express extreme behaviors such as aggression, autism, and ADHD. My friend fought for custody of her grandchildren because her son and his girlfriend were too addicted to drugs to raise them. In her 60s, at an age when she should be retiring, she was granted custody of these two children.

I don't know how she gets up every day to keep climbing this mountain. Her grandkids have extreme outbursts of behaviors that she has to constantly mediate. And on top of this, she has her own health challenges to deal with. She struggles to find the support she needs.

Coloring Outside the Lines: I take care of my friends.

I would like you to think of a friend who could use your love and support. Who do you know who could use a little extra pick-me-up?

Take the time to show your friend how amazing he or she is. This kind of compassion reflects back to you, showing you how amazing you are.

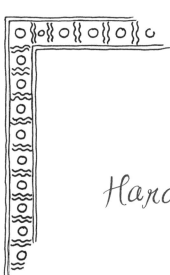

Hard Times Are for a Reason

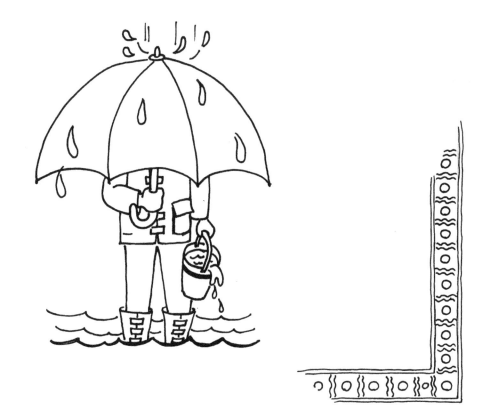

Hard Times Are for a Reason

In October of 2007 I left the Phoenix and moved to Flagstaff to start NI (naturopathsinternational.org). I opened the practice and outreach to NI and got involved in the community as soon as I could. As I got to know people, I heard repeatedly I wouldn't make it "because there was too much poverty." The locals called the area "poverty with a view". Even public radio announcers talked about Flagstaff with this phrase! Local newspapers published it.

As I heard "poverty with a view" I started to believe it. My practice and organization began to reflect this belief. I found myself not making enough money to pay my rent much less buy groceries. To survive, I found myself going homeless. I showered at a local health club, slept on the floor in a treatment room in my office, and stored my few possessions in one of the closets in my clinic. I cried myself to sleep every night for several months. I felt like a complete failure. Then my brother passed in June of 2010 in a motorcycle accident. It was such an incredible shock; there are no words to capture the pain I felt in losing him!

My situation was the worst it had ever been. Here I was a homeless, penniless physician grieving over the loss of someone very close to me. While I had no physical resources to draw upon—no friends or family where I lived to support me—I did have a tiny seed in my heart that craved life and success. It was a tiny voice! And yet, this tiny voice said I just had to climb out of my sense of depression and failure. I just had to. And somehow I knew I could, even though my physical reality looked impossible.

Because of this belief, I worked hard to follow it in spite of my external situations. I rose up out of a very bad situation, both financially and emotionally. I feel great today!

Coloring Outside the Lines: I can do anything I put my mind to.

Think of something that scares you, such as an activity that you secretly have been craving to do, but never have. How would it feel to accomplish it?

What steps would it take for you to achieve that?

Write the steps to accomplishing that which you fear here:

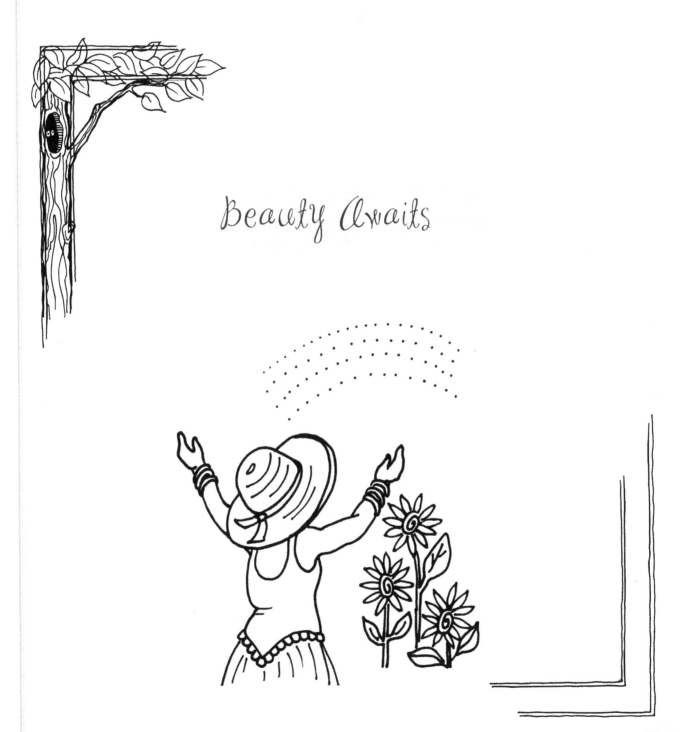

Beauty Awaits

Beauty Awaits

I hiked a stunningly beautiful area outside of Flagstaff today called the Weatherford trail. The Weatherford is a strenuous trail; climbing slowly but steadily towards Humphreys Peak at just over 12,000 feet. I hike several miles a week and am in good shape, but this day I felt fatigued; the incline of the hike pushed my physical limits.

Two hours into the hike I had several thoughts of turning around. The trail was rocky, which was hard on my legs and feet. I was sweaty and hot. I didn't bring enough water and my dog was even getting a bit overwhelmed by the heat. I stopped for a few moments to rest under the pines and gave some water to my dog. I looked up and down the trail. Up ahead the trail curved to the left, and while I was curious as to what lie ahead, I felt exhausted and was seeing all that was wrong with my situation.

As I was making myself grumpy with my thoughts, the trail leveled out and took a slight bend to the right where trees cleared, allowing for a view of the valley below. I could see Flagstaff miles off in the distance, as well as miles and miles of forest, cliffs where the forest met the desert, eagles soaring above it all, and the Humphreys Peak behind me. The sun no longer felt oppressive. The air was fresh. The wind whispered gently through the pines, the clouds billowed by. My dog and I sat to rest, sharing the last of our water. Lovely. I looked over to my dog happily sitting next to me. She enjoys beauty too.

Coloring Outside the Lines: I always see the beauty around me.

I want you to go somewhere you have either wanted to explore and haven't made time, or go somewhere you love to go. Keep your heart open to what you may see, notice, observe, think about, or discover about yourself or life. What did you discover?

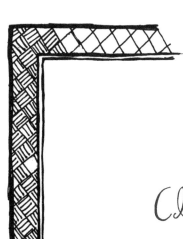

Clean the Clutter Out!

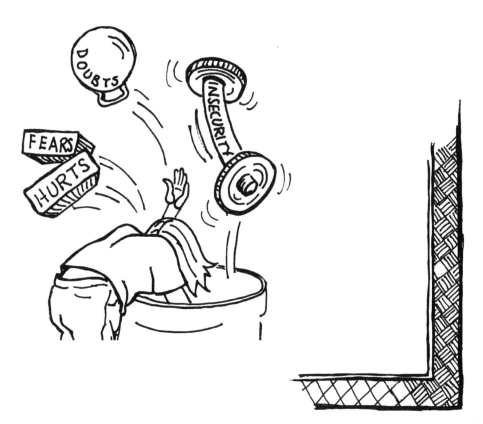

Clean the Clutter Out!

We all have too many negative junk thoughts playing around and around in our minds. Take it to the trash. Picture the Apple Mac screen in your mind. You know how there is a little trash icon at the bottom of every Mac computer screen? Put the image of the screen in your mind. When a negative, junk thought comes, imagine a cursor highlighting that thought, click on it, and drag it to the junk box. Now hear the sound the Mac makes when a piece of trash has gone in.

Take it to the trash! Life is too short to allow garbage to keep recirculating in your mind. Focusing on the positive is key for a good life.

Coloring Outside the Lines: I am a positive thinker.

Put yourself in a nice quiet place, whether that is sitting on a sunny spot in the forest, finding a quiet corner in a coffee shop, or carving out time at home. Either way, you need time for reflection without things that distract you.

Have this journal with you, and sketch out negative thoughts that tend to play over and over in your mind.

How does it make you feel to think and write down these negative thoughts?

How does it make you feel to think and write down these negative thoughts?

Now write down the exact opposite of these negative statements, things that are positive.

How does thinking and writing the positive make you feel?

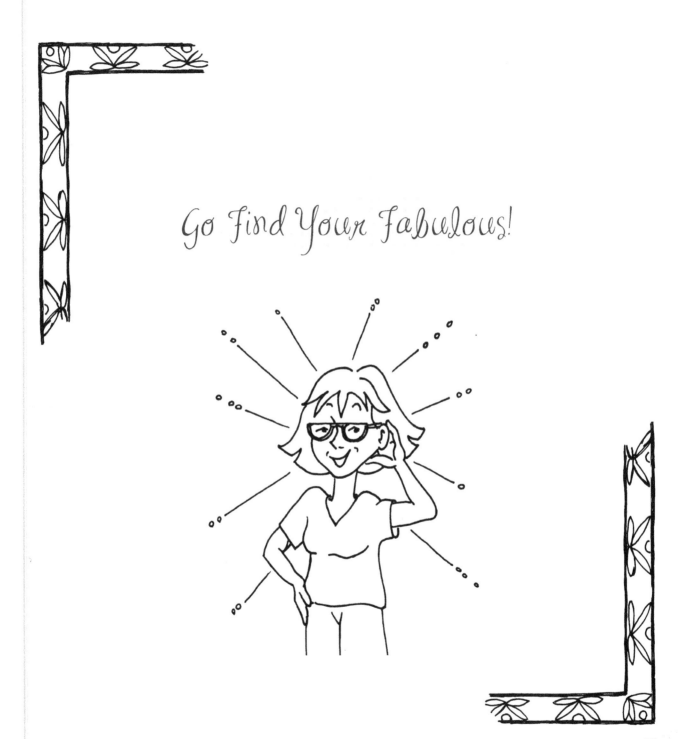

Go Find Your Fabulous!

Go Find Your Fabulous!

I have a patient struggling with life changes. Over the last several months she lost her job, her dog passed away, she broke up with the man she thought was her soulmate, and she felt forced into a lawsuit. She felt like a mess. She was trying to incorporate stress management techniques, but felt like it wasn't enough. Tears rolled as she spoke.

I listened for a while and then found myself telling her she needed to "go find her fabulous." She needed to find herself. She could only do this by continuing to move forward and not give up. I gave her a hug and told her she should start to find that fabulous by taking an inventory of good she has done and what has been wonderful in her life.

Coloring Outside the Lines: I am fabulous!

Have you taken a good look at all the good you have done in your life?

Take time to inventory your life and write a list of your accomplishments here:

How does it make you feel to look at your list of accomplishments?

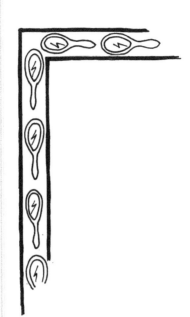

Who Are You?

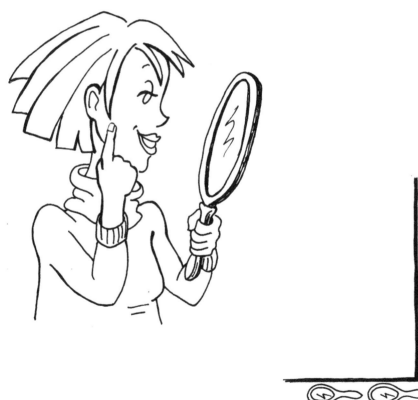

Who Are You?

I had a new patient today with a long-standing history of alcoholism (25 years). The first thing she said when she came in and sat down was that she was finally sober and she wanted to keep it that way. She told me, "I'm ready to change my life." During the history taking, I asked her what was going on in her life when she first started to drink. She shared that many life changes hit at the same time and it overwhelmed her. So she turned to alcohol to help her cope, but she no longer wanted to use it as a crutch. She wanted to find herself and develop that as her strength rather than use alcohol as her strength.

Coloring Outside the Lines: I know who I am.

A lot of us define ourselves by what we do or children we raise. We rarely look past that into who we really are at our core. How do we begin to answer that question? One way is to explore the way we feel when we are doing a favorite activity. What is your favorite activity? Drawing? Dancing? Doing an art project? Going for a walk?

Think about how you feel when you do these things and write them here:

These feelings are part of who you are. Explore them deeply to learn more about your deepest self.

What did you learn about who you are?

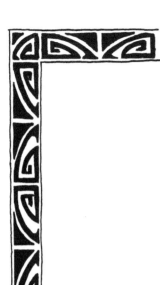

I Follow My Joy

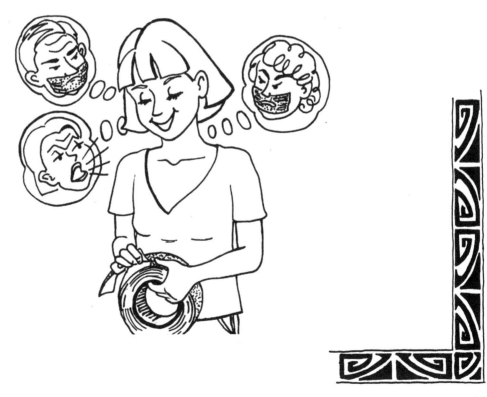

I Follow My Joy

One of my patients came to me the other day to discuss her ongoing health challenges. During the course of the visit, I realized she was unhappy and sick because she wasn't doing things she wanted. She felt she needed to be traveling and visiting loved ones, but had not been going anywhere lately. I asked her why and her response was a too-familiar phrase:

"My husband won't let me…"

Ladies, the only one not letting you do something is **you**.

Coloring Outside the Lines: I follow my joy.

Too many let others tell them how to live. I think this is a mistake. If you let others tell you how to live, you could end up making yourself sick. I imagine that when you allow someone else to tell you what to do, how to think, or how to be, there is something on the inside of you that rebels against that.

There is no time like the present moment, and really, no time to waste following someone else's joy. You have to live from your joy. What path are you not following that you know you should be?

What can you do differently to follow your joy?

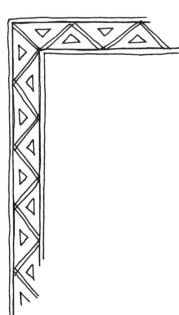

Women Know

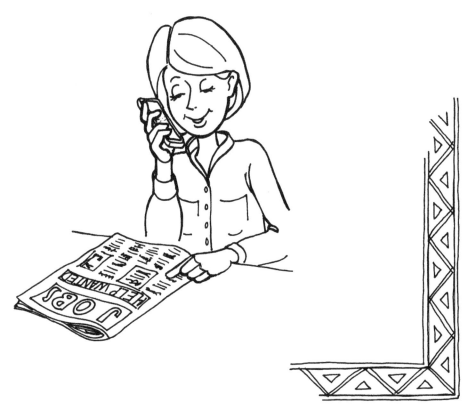

Women Know

Women have an intuition about partners and children that can be very powerful. We know who our partners are as soon as we meet them. We know the names of our children and their personalities before they're born. We know the next steps to take in our lives.

Coloring Outside the Lines: I trust my intuition.

I have learned that the more I trust my instinct and follow it, the better my life gets.

What has been nagging you deep in the pit of your stomach? perhaps something you know you should do but have been ignoring.

Why do you think you have been ignoring this instinct?

How would it feel to you to follow your intuition?

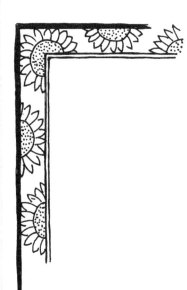

Accepting Yourself the Way You Are

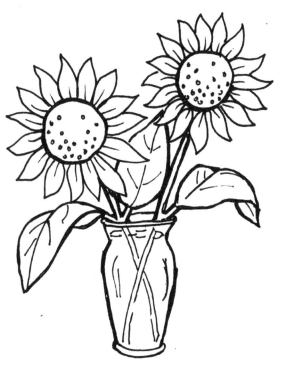

Accepting Yourself the Way You Are

Women spend so much money trying to be "perfect" like models and superstars on magazine covers. Your body is perfect the way it is.

Coloring Outside the Lines: I am perfect the way I am.

Is your attention easily captured by beautiful things, people, places, or objects? If so, then you are beautiful, too! You cannot see something and appreciate it unless it is also a quality you possess.

I would like you to purchase a small bouquet of flowers for yourself. Any kind that you love. Bring them home, and when you are alone sit in meditation and allow your eyes to rest on those flowers.

What do you notice about the flowers? The vibrant color? The wonderful odor? The shapeliness to the curve of the petals? The texture of the petals when you reach out to feel them? You are just as perfect as these flowers are.

All these sensations, colors, and feelings of these flowers are all the amazing things about you. Allow yourself time to enjoy the experience! Take your time with this activity. What did you learn about yourself?

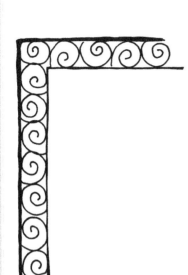

Sometimes You Need to Rest

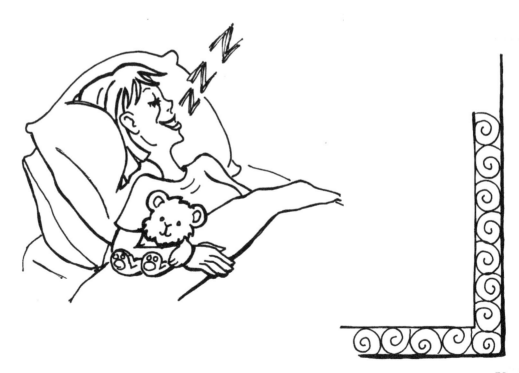

Sometimes You Need to Rest

Life is oftentimes overwhelming. Someone always needs us: our projects, our children, our pets, our mothers, our fathers, our partners, our friends, our co-workers, our work. I wish I could give more of myself without becoming exhausted but this is not possible—we all need rest. I do need that time where I don't answer the phone or respond to emails. I have to take that time to rest and take time to nurse my spirit.

Coloring Outside the Lines: I rest when I need to.

We tend to put ourselves on the back-burner. I can't tell you how many women I have had come to my office for acupuncture whom I have to gently tell to stop talking about their friends or family for just 30 minutes while they rest with the treatment. It is key to rest so that we do not get burned out on life or those we love.

I would like you to practice the art of daily rest. If it is yoga that gives you rest, do a little every day. If it is drawing or playing music, make sure you devote yourself to it regularly.

What do you love that gives you rest?

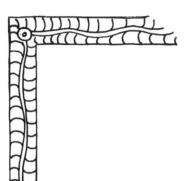

Be in Your Dream

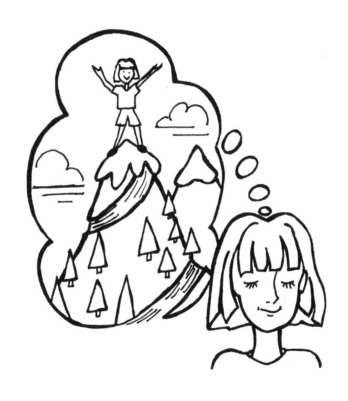

Be in Your Dream

You have to be in the energetic space of what you feel needs to be your life before it can come to pass. Nothing can come into physical being without the energetic blueprint first, and this is not something you can force. Manifestation is also timing-related; if it is not time in the big scheme of things (from a universal perspective), then it is not time, and no matter how hard you try nothing will come. You have to wait and be your best where you are until you feel the energy that it is time. While you are waiting, you need to do what you can to help things along while you keep a good attitude and stay in faith.

Coloring Outside the Lines:
I am patient while my dreams come to pass.

I would like you to practice using meditation to put yourself in your dream. Get in a comfortable meditative space and imagine your life as it is for a few moments. Then start to visualize what your dream looks like. Take the image of your dream and transpose it over the image of what your life looks like now. Feel the energy and emotions associated with that dream image and focus on that. How does this make you feel? Excited? Joyful? Expectant? Focusing on these feelings and emotions will help you pull into existence your dream.

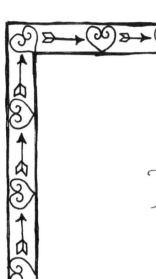

There is Nothing Better
than a Good Friend

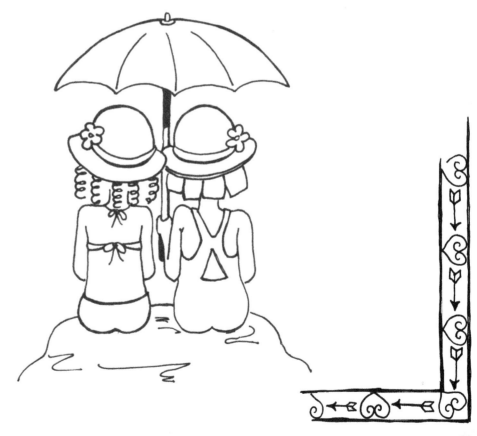

There is Nothing Better than A Good Friend

I don't know how I could have gotten to where I am without my friends. A good friend is invaluable, worth more than all the money in the world. There is nothing better to me than taking time out to spend time with a good friend. In that space of friendship, I find a safe space for expressing myself—my feelings, desires, and dreams.

Coloring Outside the Lines: I value my friendships.

It is easy to lose track of time. Moments go by so quickly, that if we are not mindful of how we use our time, before we know it, another week has gone by. Do any of us really take the time to show our friends how much they mean to us? Think about one of your closest friends. I would like you to think about what your friend really likes to do (perhaps go to the movies or dinner) and design a Date Night just for them. Get dressed up and take your friend out!

What was this experience like?

Sometimes You Have to
Dance Around in Your
Living Room, Naked,
to Loud Music,
Under the Moon

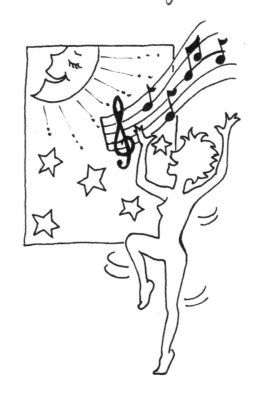

65

Sometimes You Have to Dance Around in Your Living Room, Naked, to Loud Music, Under the Moon

You know what I am talking about.

Don't deny yourself that time…and space.

Coloring Outside the Lines:
I live in joy by expressing myself physically.

Movement is one of the best ways to connect to your body. Connecting to your body creates joy. Ballroom dancers are the happiest people I know! What kind of movement brings you joy? Dancing? Yoga? Hiking? Whatever it is, write about how it makes you feel, and then go do it! Make sure you are doing this activity on a weekly basis.

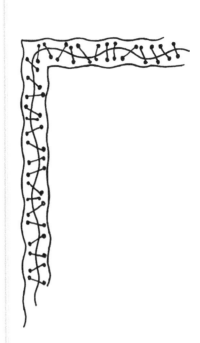

Don't Worry!

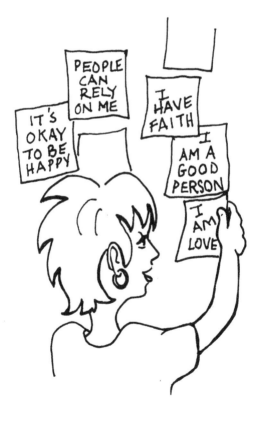

Don't Worry!

We all worry because life can be so stressful; but I see that worry gives women wrinkles, so try not to worry! Here is my anti-aging secret prescription for you: Stop worrying! I have heard that Abraham Hicks says, "Worry creates the future we don't want." Other sages say we create our outcomes; be careful not to project what you don't want, as it may come true.

Coloring Outside the Lines: I always trust.

What do you worry about? How does this make you feel?

Now contemplate what the opposites are to your worry statements. For example, if you worry about money, the opposite would be, "I have lots of money."

For every worry statement you have in your mind, write down the opposite below:

Now take all the fearless statements and write them on pieces of paper. Post the pieces all over your home in places you will easily see them. Keep the pieces of paper up for you to see until the worry thoughts start to diminish, and your mind is flooded only with the positive such as, "I have lots of money." You have to have faith in these positive things first for them to become a reality. It takes time to shift your thinking, but if you persist with it, it will happen for you.

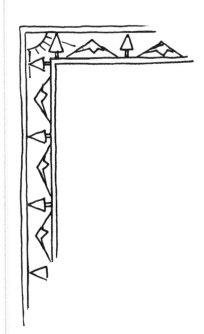

Time Alone

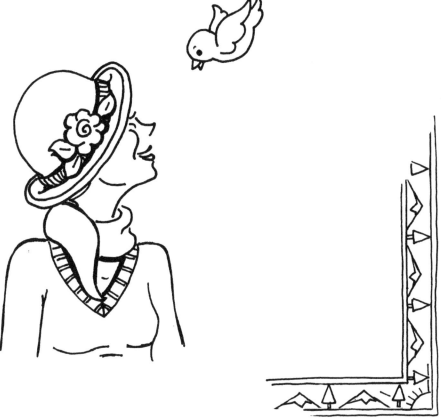

Time Alone

Being willing to spend time alone takes strength and courage. When I work with patients on getting them off their medications, they often tell me they feel "cracked open." The meds were covering up how they really felt and now that those chemicals are working their way out of the body, the original emotional pain rears up. Stay brave, and go deep into it—slowly, if you need to.

Alone time is a blessing, not a curse. Savor it because life changes continually. You may suddenly find yourself with a partner and kids with limited time to yourself! Savor alone time while you have it; and if you don't have it, try to find ways to carve out that alone time.

Coloring Outside the Lines: I enjoy my alone time.

I would just like you to go for a walk by yourself. Pick a neighborhood, park, or hiking trail you have not been to. Get yourself dressed appropriately for a nice walk and leave your cell phone at home. Spend at least 30 minutes walking solo, and pay attention to your thoughts and feelings. Do you feel tense initially, worried, or scared? Note these thoughts and feelings. Then notice how it feels to just be with you.

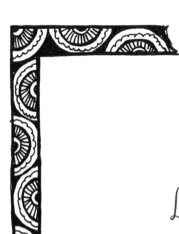

Life Is in the Moment

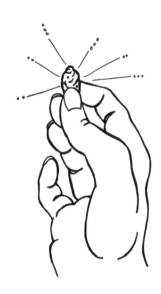

Life Is in the Moment

I think this is something that dogs are really good at doing.

My dog is incredible. She's always in the moment. She never seems to look back or forward, knows what she wants, and is always loving. It is so much fun when I take her hiking! She has an expression of joy on her face that's amazing to see! She runs, sniffs plants, and chases squirrels. She is in the moment, loving every second of life!

Coloring Outside the Lines: I live in the moment.

Years ago I took a mindfulness meditation course. We did an activity whereby we were given a single raisin and asked to chew it slowly over a minute. What did we notice? I noticed how wonderful that raisin tasted and seemed to have various layers of sweet taste as I chewed. This experience was very interesting and put me in the moment.

Practice an activity such as this. Perhaps sip a cup of coffee or tea slowly to put yourself in the moment. What do you notice?

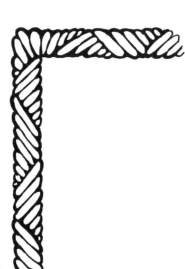

Nourish Your Body

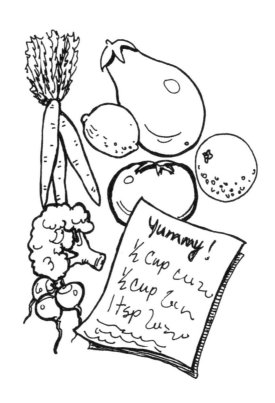

Nourish Your Body

My experience in working with my patients is that processed foods contribute to an incredible array of diseases, from anxiety to cancer or autoimmune diseases. When I recommend patients go off of processed sugars and they follow through with it, I see huge shifts in their disease processes. People with MS start to see a decrease in neurological symptoms. Patients with cancer start to develop the ability to overcome cancer. Patients with depression start to feel happier. Those who can't sleep start to feel sleepy at night. Or, patients with arthritis notice a decrease in joint pain.

Coloring Outside the Lines:
I nourish my body with wholesome foods.

Changing your diet is not easy, but it is possible. My patients trust me when I recommend starting a sugar-abstinence diet. It starts with taking stock of what is currently in your refrigerator and pantry.

Make a list here of the foods you currently have that are either processed (i.e. breads, pastas) or have added sugars in the ingredient list, such as glycerin, corn syrup, fructose, honey, agave nectar, or sugar itself.

Make your list here:

Now make a list of the foods you have in your refrigerator or pantry that are *not processed* or *do not have extra sugars* added.

Is your diet overwhelmed with the foods that are processed/sugary? Start to switch out these foods for whole-food items. Make sure you read labels in grocery stores. If it has added sugars, don't buy it. The next time you go shopping, can you fill your cart with whole-food items, ones you actually have to cook? What are the colors of these items? Bright? Bright foods are the best as they have the most nutrients and antioxidants.

Find a whole-food recipe (a recipe with no processed foods) that you want to try, and write it here:

Make this special recipe and try it! How did the nourishing food make you feel?

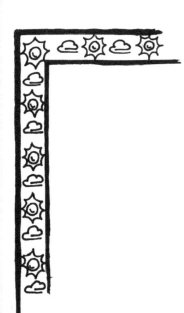

Life Is Good

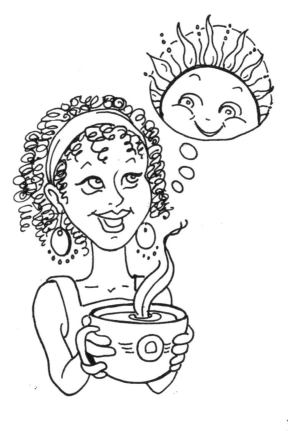

Life Is Good

"Life is Hard, Dr. B," one of my patients told me the other day as I was getting her situated for her acupuncture treatment. She has had so many struggles and hardships in her life.

Life can be very challenging—I am not going to deny that.

Let's examine together ways it can be very difficult:

Financial Challenges   Difficulty Staying Positive-minded

Addictions   Abuse   Trauma   PTSD   Stress

Physical Limitations   Chronic Disease   Learning Disabilities

Feeling like you're not in a place in life that you want to be

In contrast, lets look at what makes life good:

Time in Nature	Family	Holidays
Love	Children	Beauty
Good Food	Good Books	Pets
Travel	Good Restaurants	Faith
Friends	Summertime	Exercise

The ability to exercise at a nice workout facility

Coloring Outside the Lines: I focus on the good in my life.

I do not want to put down anyone's experiences, but I do want to remind you to look for the good. I understand it can be a struggle to look for the good—especially if you have lived through extremely hard circumstances.

I work with a lot of patients who have been (or are experiencing) very challenging times. But we can choose to rise above the negative situations and move our lives into places of peace, abundance, and gratitude.

You have to be willing to do the work and not be afraid to look deep into your heart. You have to be willing to admit what has hurt you, and willing to do something about it. You have to be willing to face the pain and move through it into the place you really want to be emotionally. This takes a lot of strength and vulnerability.

I want you to spend a few hours thinking only about what is good. No negative thoughts. Take yourself out to your favorite coffee shop and think about the good in your life!

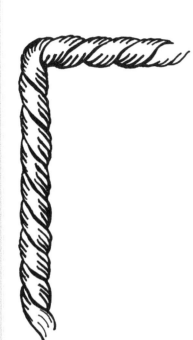

Let Go

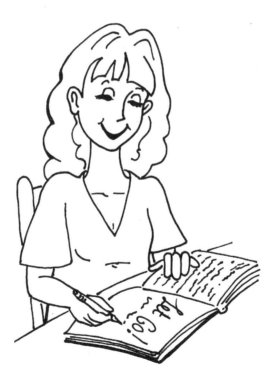

Let Go

When I was 20 I met a man I would marry. We started to spend a lot of time together and I fell hard! He was the one who introduced me to natural foods, tea, and the joy of camping. Without him I was a pack-a-gallon-jug-of-water-and-some-beef-jerky-in-a-backpack-and-go-hiking kind of girl. I was a bit behind the times and rustic. I got my first official backpack from him, as well as a camping pad. Wow, a camping pad, who invented that! We had great adventures!

After a few years we got married. Four years later we divorced.

From this experience I learned to know when it was time to let someone go.

Coloring Outside the Lines: I let go.

Letting go is not easy. But even more important and difficult is knowing when to let go of our ideas of what our life is to be. If anyone would have told me I would end up divorcing this man I would have laughed in their face, and yet here I am, years later, single. If anyone would have told me I would be in medical school I would have laughed in disbelief, and yet here I am, years later, running a non-profit medical practice. If I didn't let go when I did, at places in my life that I felt a shift needed to occur, I would not be where I am today.

You have to learn to let go when it is time to do so. I would like you to set aside time to reflect where things are in your life currently. Is there something you need to make a change to, to let go of? No matter how simple or complex that question may be, please take time to think this over. I want you to do this activity in your PJ's: go make a nice cup of hot tea, climb into your favorite PJs, and then journal here what you need to let go of. Don't censor your thoughts.

Write whatever comes to mind here:

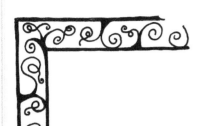

Remember to be Pursued, Not to Pursue!

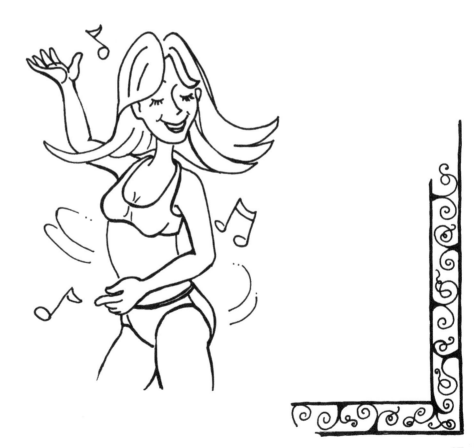

Remember to be Pursued, Not to Pursue!

Discover how to get so lost in God that a guy has to seek Him to find you.
—Dannah Gresh

This quote was on the back cover of a book I had gotten in the mail, and I'm not actually sure how I got the book or who sent it to me. The title of the book was **Get Lost** and has a picture of a woman sitting alone on a tree trunk, with a rose next to her on the tree. She is gazing out into a field of green with beautiful trees in the background. She looks peaceful; as though she has found her place and is sitting quietly in that space.

I'm not sure what exactly that quote touched on the inside of me other than it resonated. After being through a divorce, thinking so-and-so's are "my soulmates", and working on my self-esteem for well over forever, I think I was ready for that quote.

We have a hard time letting ourselves be pursued. But pursued we must let ourselves be…but not until we know what is in our heart.

According to Stasi Eldredge who authored the book *Captivating* with her husband John,

…the heart is central. "Above all else, guard your heart, for it is the wellspring of life" (Prov. 4:23). Above all else. Why? Because God knows that our heart is core to who we are. It is the source of all our creativity, our courage, and our convictions. It is the fountainhead of our faith, our hope, and of course, our love. This "wellspring of life" within us is the very essence of our existence, the center of our being. Your heart as a women is the most important thing about you.

Think about it: God created you as a woman. "God created man in his own image…male and female he created them" (Gen. 1:27). Whatever it means to bear God's image, you do so as a woman. Female. That's how and where you bear his image. Your feminine heart has been created with the greatest of all possible dignities—as a reflection of God's own heart. You are a woman to your soul, to the very core of your being…

Now look at what John says is at the core of a man/male energy:

…there are three core desires in the heart of every man…every man wants a battle to fight. It's the whole thing with boys and weapons…men also long for adventure. Boys love to climb and jump and see how fast they can ride their bikes (with no hands). Just look in your garage—all the gear and go-carts and motorcycles and ropes and boats and stuff. This isn't about "boys and their toys." Adventure is a deeply spiritual longing in the heart of every man. Adventure requires something of us, puts us to the test.

Finally, every man longs for a Beauty to rescue. He really does…you see, it is not just that a man needs a battle to fight. He needs someone to fight for.

If our heart rests quietly, then a man/male energy would be pulled into that energy and in that pulling would find him/herself on a deeper level. We have to hold the space so that can happen for our partners.

Coloring Outside the Lines: I sit still in my heart.

Whether you are married, single, or dating, the same truth runs true for all women: we need to sit still in our hearts. We need to sit still so that we can see what is trying *to come into our lives*, whether that be a partner or something completely unrelated. Either way, the energies of the universe, if we let them, pursue us, not the other way around. If we stay still, we can see what is coming!

The idea of sitting still can apply to all aspects of our life, not just in the discussion of partners. You need to sit still while you wait for dreams to come to pass…for children to be born…for goals to be met!

Dance is a way to put yourself in that stillness. You can be moving but your heart can be still. Try this. When you are alone, put on some comfortable clothing and play music you love. Allow your body to move to the music. There are no rules with how you should move, just move. As you move, thoughts should drift away and your mind will automatically be in the present moment. This is your stillness.

How did this experience make you feel?

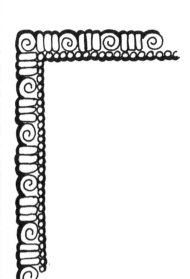

Soulmates?

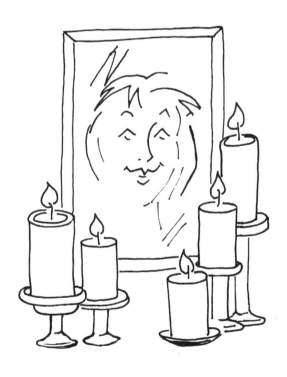

Soulmates?

The movies tell us "I found the One", I "am looking for the One", or "I can't live without the One". What if the "One" we were really looking for is our *self*?

I was watching a movie called ***Lola Versus*** which made me think of the topic of this essay. If you have not seen this movie, rent it. It is about a woman who has a hard breakup; then obsesses over the breakup for a year. She obsesses over other men and keeps trying to fill the void in her life she felt from the absence of a man in it. In the end, however, she realizes all she really needs is herself.

She has learned that the real "One" is our *self!*

You are the One. You are all you need, really. Anyone else is a bonus. People complement our life and make it better, but we can do for ourselves. I love the end of this movie. The actress the movie was following is shown buying herself a bouquet of flowers and then going home to a quiet house. She sits down at her kitchen table and looks around her apartment with complete contentment. You get the idea that the life she has, she created. She realizes she created it, she is happy to be creating it, and she wants more of that.

Coloring Outside the Lines: I am all I need.

Relationships are important, but the relationship you have with yourself is the most important.

For this activity, I want you to first go scrub clean your bathroom. Then go get some candles and light them all over that shiny clean bathroom. Make sure the lighting is good by your mirror. Now take a deep breath, and yes, stare at yourself. What do you see? Do you see your nose, eyes, or maybe what you are wearing? What else do you see?

Now look deeper. Take your time. Really look. What else do you see? Do you see someone capable of raising children, running a business, or writing a book? Do you see someone who caregives for aging parents or siblings? Do you see someone who took their company to a new level, or just completed a degree? Whatever you see, write it here:

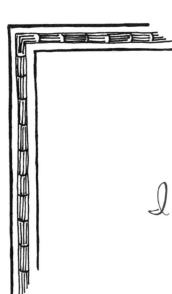

I Am My Best Partner

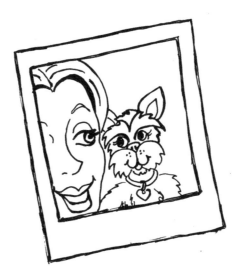

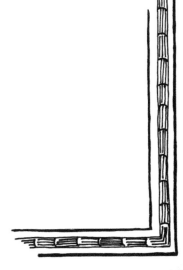

I Am My Best Partner

Recently, I experienced a moment of alignment with another living being as I was biking. A few days a week I bike to my office and I always take my dog with me. She has been by my side for years helping me see patients. She is amazing with my patients. Very sweet!

On the bike ride home, there is a mile stretch of road that is usually quiet and free of traffic, so I let her run beside me without a leash. She loves this time! That day, she ran in line with my bike and speed; we were in perfect unison and synchronicity. I could feel our energies joined, lined up, synced, together. She ran forward blissfully, looking over at me occasionally with a huge grin on her face. Her steps were in alignment with my peddling. She never went ahead of me or fell behind. I think even our breathing matched!

This made me think about partners in life. As women, we assume a partner means a romantic life partner. Movies and other forms of media teach this to us. But I think we can have any type of partner who gives us a lot of love and support. A partner doesn't have to be someone we marry or live with.

Coloring Outside the Lines: I am open to partners of all kinds.

You really are your best partner. Have you ever thought of life in this term? Or in this way? My dad always used to tell me that I was all I needed, and I never really understood that until I got older and experienced enough life to realize how right he was. No one can make me happy except me. I have to generate this kind of Chi from within my heart. You can do this too. How does thinking of life from this perspective make you feel?

I Stay in My Joy

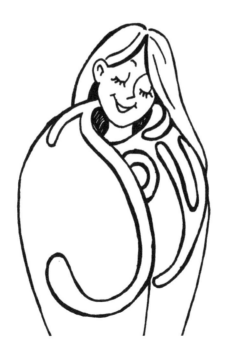

I Stay in My Joy

Dogs are good at staying in their joy. My dog's favorite activity is hiking. If it means the promise of an adventure and exploration, she is first in line.

She is so fun to watch on the trail. She is in the moment with a fun little prance as she walks; her ears flopping to her cadence. I swear she smiles a big grin when we are out.

Children are also good at being in their joy. I have a three-year-old patient who is so adorable when she comes into my office in her little tutu. She twirls with joy to show it off! We all would do so much better in life if we spent more time enjoying things rather than complaining. We all start out as one of those in-the-moment little beings! Maybe we can focus on going back to that kind of place once in a while?

Coloring Outside the Lines: My life is a joyful experience!

What brings you joy? What do you like to focus your love on? Focusing on what you love can bring you into your joy!

Think about what you love to do. Is that painting a portrait? Or maybe singing a song? Dancing? Or do you love your work?

Now get out those paintbrushes, or your music, or your work, whatever it is you love. Carve out the time whereby you can focus 100% on whatever it is that you love. Focus entirely on it. Put your mind in the present moment. Now, what do you notice? How do you feel when you put your focus on what you love? Does it bring you joy?

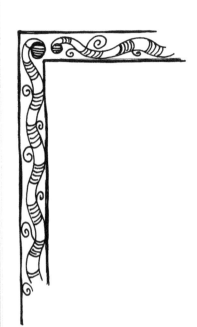

Appreciation!

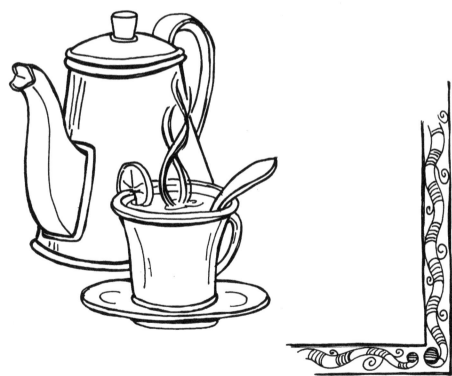

Appreciation!

We don't spend enough time enjoying our lives. We miss the little things all the time as we rush around running errands, or hurrying to make dinner. Why is this? Who taught us that we need to rush? When we rush we miss the moments that make life so good.

Coloring Outside the Lines: I appreciate every moment of my life.

I think tea-time is important; and I am not talking about your rush to the coffee shop to grab a beverage on the way to work. I am talking about the deliberate action of brewing up the water for tea and steeping your favorite tea in your favorite cup. While taking a few minutes to enjoy it. Sip it slowly…smell the vapors of tea coming off the steam. Try this, every day.

What do you notice?

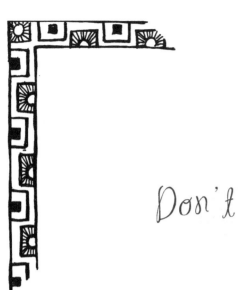

Don't Let Moments Pass

Don't Let Moments Pass

I did a road trip once from Flagstaff towards Denver for a conference where I took all back roads to get there. A few hundred miles into the trip, I got struck by most of the words that became this book. The words were flowing so fast that I dictated as I drove. Later, when I went to type the words, I was amazed at how little editing it needed.

There was one chapter I got the idea for while on a hike outside Breckenridge. I didn't have pen and paper with me at the time, but I thought it was such a great idea how could I possibly forget it? I had my cell phone with me and could have dictated the words but I didn't. I decided of course I would remember such a juicy book chapter! But alas, by the time I got back to my car I had completely forgotten what I was supposed to write about.

This means there is an essay in this journal that never got written.

Coloring Outside the Lines: I always seize the moment.

For the next few days, I want you to stay very open to events and moments that happen around you. Is there a moment to seize?

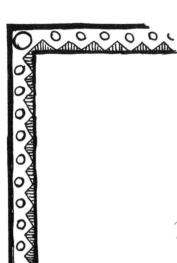

Sometimes a Girl Has to Hit the Road

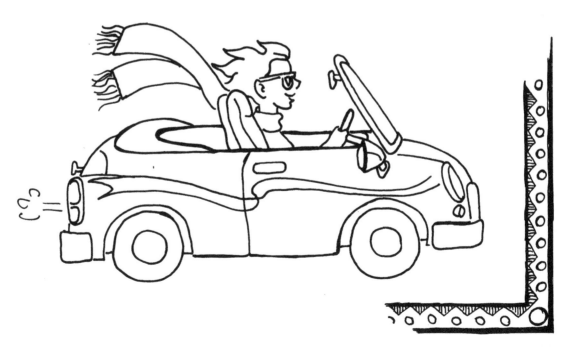

Sometimes a Girl Has to Hit the Road

We all have ways to keep balance. For me it's going on solo road trips. I can feel when I have worked too much, gave too much to my patients, gave too much to my work, didn't sleep enough, or didn't play enough. I get grouchy. No one needs a grouchy friend or doctor. It is my responsibility to take the best care of myself that I can. No one else can do this for me.

The best thing for me is hitting the road. It doesn't matter where I go or when, as long as I am away for several days at a time. If I go with others I feel like my style gets cramped, so I learned a long time ago the virtues of solo travel. A lot of women are afraid to hit the road by themselves—even though secretly they want to. Doesn't that sound so blissful? A few days all to yourself, no one to ask you questions, no one to ask you to do things, no one to ask you to help them, no one asking anything! The most complicated question you may get is when you stop at a gas station for some road travel treats and the cashier says, "Will that be all?"

Coloring Outside the Lines: I love to try new things!

Hit the road! See what is out there. Get out of your comfort zone. You will most likely see yourself shift in ways you did not fathom. Take this journal when you go!

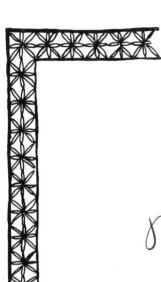

Life is Too Short Not to Wear Cute Shoes

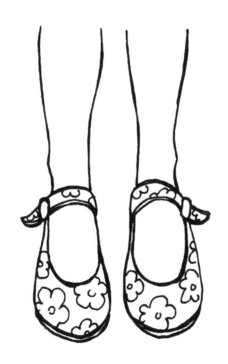

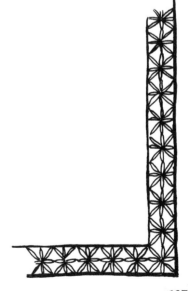

Life is Too Short Not to Wear Cute Shoes

This was said to me by one of my regular patients. She saw the cowgirl boots I was wearing, and was surprised to see a physician wear their boots to work. I told her, "If I felt like if I wanted to wear the boots, why not?" She thought about it a moment and then exclaimed, "Life is too short not to wear cute shoes!"

Coloring Outside the Lines: I love to express myself!

What is your favorite article of clothing, piece of jewelry or pair of shoes to wear? Do you stop yourself from wearing any of these because you worry about what others may think? Why do you worry about what others may think?

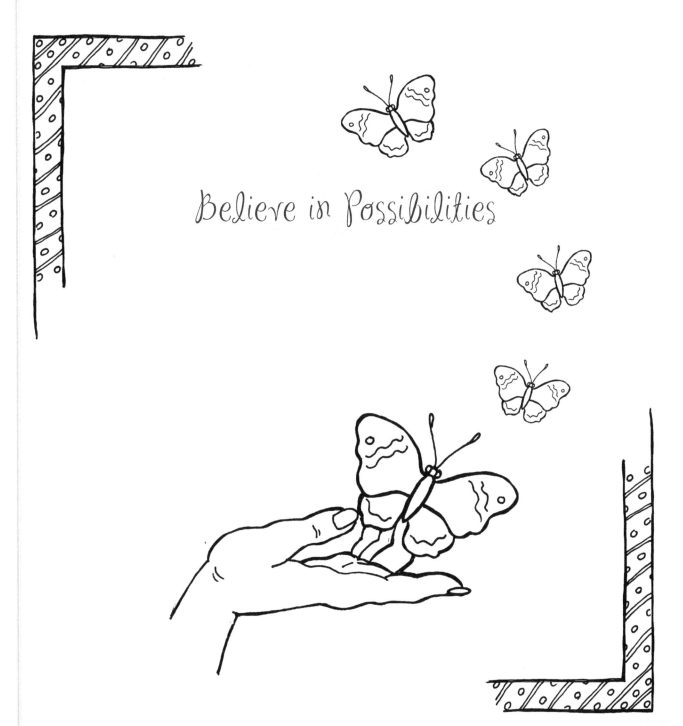

Believe in Possibilities

Believe in Possibilities

Too many of us today don't believe in or look for possibilities. We live in the past, we live in the future, or we don't live at all. We expect others to take care of us. We expect life to be easy. It is not easy. But life should be seen as an adventure full of possibilities!

Coloring Outside the Lines: I believe my life is full of possibilities.

How do you look at your life? As something you have to do or as something that is full of possibilities and adventure? How you see your life determines your day.

I want you to try changing how you view your life, starting with your thoughts in the morning. Train yourself to say to yourself as soon as you wake, "Today is going to be magical." Then as you go through your day, stay mindful to the little things that make your day good. The "magic" of life doesn't have to be anything big, or even extraordinary. It just has to be good. In my opinion, goodness is the magic.

What did you notice?

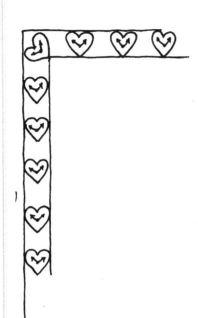

The Gift of Time

The Gift of Time

There is nothing better you can give someone than your time, your talents, and your energy.

When you look back on your life what is it that you remember? Things you got or people you knew? Adventures you went on?

Coloring Outside the Lines: I see life as a gift.

Early in my career, I was present at the passing of one of my patients. He had actually been a new patient whose wife brought him to me for palliative care. He was dying of liver cancer. With the help of a cardiologist I work with in the coordination of patient care, we got him admitted to the hospital for his last days. I won't ever, ever forget the last moments of his life. He was coming in and out of consciousness. His wife sat close to him on the hospital bed, and when he came back into consciousness his words and memories were so clear. He wasn't talking about things they bought together in their 30 years of marriage. He was taking the time he had left to tell her that he loved her, that he was grateful for their time, and he wanted her to keep living and enjoying her life. It was such a beautiful thing to witness. Sad, but beautiful at the same time.

Practice carving out time to spend with someone you care about. Don't plan any activity other than sitting down with them and asking how they are. Maybe brew up a nice cup of coffee or tea and sit down to chat. Don't make this time about you at all. Only ask them how they are, and really listen.

What did you learn from this experience?

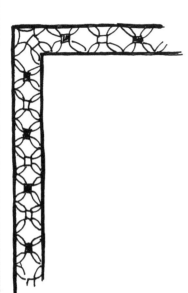

Be Mindful

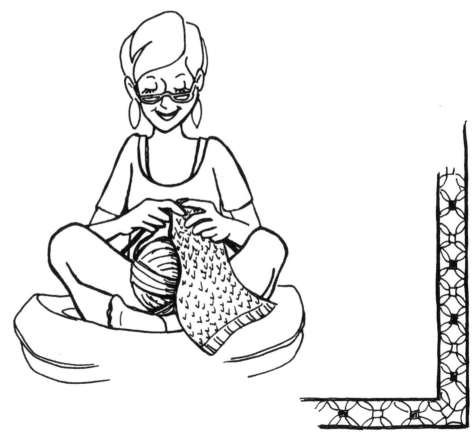

Be Mindful

For the mindfulness discussion, I am going to divert the discussion of the topic to an associate, Nicolette Sachs, a Licensed Social Worker in private practice in Flagstaff:

A dear friend invited me to go on retreat in San Diego led by a Zen Buddhist Monk and his followers. At that time, I had not had much exposure to meditation or Buddhist teachings; certainly not in a purposeful way. The Monk's name is Thich Nhat Hanh. Although I'd never seen his photo, the night before we left for retreat I dreamt of him, my unconscious mind depicting him accurately. I took this as a sign that I was on the right path. The retreat was a wonderful experience. I felt an inner glow, a softness encircling my heart, when I first heard Thich Nhat Hanh (Thay as his followers call him) give a Dharma talk. It felt like coming home. The Monks and Nuns seemed to float around the grounds with a half-smile on their faces. "What did they know that I didn't?" I wondered. They sang Vietnamese chants for us. With that retreat, I began a formal mindfulness practice that has done much to sustain me over the past 14 years.

Returning home from a retreat can feel brutal. For one thing, life on retreat is slower, without much distraction. This quote by Merijane Block gives pause to our tendency to hurry through life: "Everything takes longer than you think it should or thought it would, except your life." Following retreat, it's easy to feel like everyone and everything should have changed, like you believe you did, while you were away. Often though, the people you return to have not changed, and whatever conflicts or dilemmas you had when you left are there to be addressed. I saw how necessary it was for me to take my new knowledge into my life, so I worked for the next 14 years to integrate mindfulness practice into all the aspects of my life—both personal and professional. Little by little, I have become able to respond to challenging situations and stressors rather than react and realize change starts with me. Being mindful has allowed me to see this; and to recognize the importance of "being" rather than always "doing."

Stay in the moment! You never know the good it can bring your life!

Also from Nicolette,

Practicing psychotherapy as a Licensed Clinical Social Worker for over two decades has allowed me to work with many women who are trying to improve their lives. One consistent theme has been empowerment. Many women in our culture tend to sacrifice their own needs and wants for those of significant others. Convincing women to see the importance of self-nurturance and self-compassion can be challenging. Many see this as selfishness, often laden with guilt. It is so important to refresh oneself in order to then have some reserves to offer others.

The women's movement helped a lot, but there's still much progress to make. Now, it's common for women to feel like they need to work, parent, and care for a home with perfection. Negotiating roles with a partner with mutual respect and compassion is tricky. Discussions can easily erode into power struggles where one or both partners feel unsafe and invalidated.

Ours is a culture of "not enoughness", of wanting more. We tend to crave immediate gratification and this carries over to relationships. There can be a strong tendency to believe we deserve high levels of external confirmation and pleasure at every turn. It follows that it is easy to have very high expectations of partners, and if these are not met, to blame and look for someone new. How much easier it can seem to walk away and start fresh rather than stay and work toward healing! Often however, the same issues continue to arise in new relationships until one teases apart the tapestry of dynamics and builds a foundation of self-love and appreciation. Building such a foundation takes courage and tenacity. Changing lifelong habits is challenging. It can mean risking disapproval from those one cares about most. It can also feel odd and difficult to begin thinking and behaving differently from how one has always done it in the past; like paddling up stream (without a paddle). For many, depending on the degree of past challenges and personal resources, this is not short-term work. It is vulnerable work and takes time, patience, and openness with a trusted professional. As Marcel Proust wrote, "The real voyage of discovery consists not in seeking new landscapes, but in having new eyes."

Here are some discoveries made through working with women, which remains a privilege for me:

Women are strong and often unaware of their strength.

Women are loving and often exclude themselves from their love.

Women are generous. Sometimes they invest in people who don't appreciate them.

Women can be very creative. This helps them connect and expand their inner knowing.

Women can contend with much adversity, especially when they have support from family & friends.

Faith in some universal power or path offers a valuable sense of connectedness.

Women are nurturing and open. Open heartedness must include setting limits to maintain health and balance.

It can be difficult to ask for help, which leads to isolation. Reaching out for support and connection can help break the bonds of secrecy and shame.

Many women shoulder a lot of responsibility and obligations in their lives. Doing even small things out of want rather than simply need can impact one's sense of inner freedom.

It is challenging to break lifelong habits, ways of doing. Insight into one's own destructive/obstructive patterns is important. Spending time simply "being" has value. This leads to awareness, which can lead to change. Mindfulness practice is useful in this pursuit and has helped many women reconnect with their wise heart.

The need to step out of our own way and listen with open-hearted wisdom to our true self and that of others is supported in this quote by Martha Graham, the gifted choreographer: "There is a vitality, a life force that is translated through you into action. And because there is only one of you in all time, this expression is unique, and if you block it, it will never exist through any other medium and be lost."

Coloring Outside the Lines: I live in the moment.

You don't have to sit in a Lotus pose to practice or experience mindfulness. You can make this a part of your everyday experience. Think of an activity that puts your mind in the moment, whereby you are not thinking of anything except that which you are doing.

What is this activity and how does your body feel when you are focused on this? Relaxed? Peaceful?

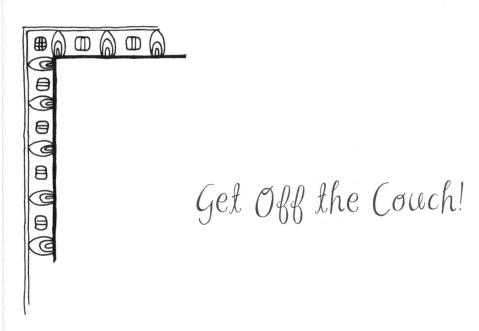

Get Off the Couch!

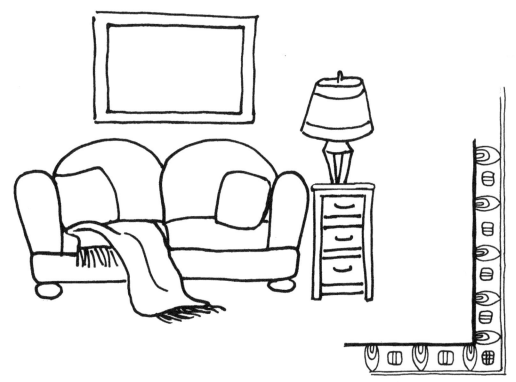

Get Off the Couch!

I am a very active person, always have been. Hiking, biking, weight lifting, yoga, and dance are a few of my favorites. I get out and do a big hike every week! I started to take line dance lessons four years ago from a great instructor, and have to say the class is one of the joys of my life.

I never thought that I would feel healthier as I got older, but I do, and I credit my activities and overall healthy lifestyle for this! My dance teacher has always made exercise part of her joy and she always has made time for it in her life. That helped her create balance. With the maintenance of balance, she always felt she had energy to then give to her family. Here are her words:

> *Ever since a young girl, dance has motivated me. At the early age of six, my mother put me in tap-dance and it made me so happy! This taught me that dance should always be a part of my life—something I could and should do forever. I knew in my heart how important dance was to me, so tap led to trying many different styles of dance, to dance recitals, and various performances. My teachers were always very encouraging and from this experience my personality and creativity shined through!*
>
> *Before I married, my husband-to-be got to see how important dance was to me. He supported me in it after we married, and still to this day! He knew as long as I was able, I would always dance. I encouraged our children to take dance lessons at a young age, and as they got older, I started to teach classes. I have been dancing for over 50 years, and I encourage you to find what you love and always do it. Don't let anything stop you, and don't waste your time sitting on the couch! Get up and move and make the time to do so!* —AF, Flagstaff, AZ

Coloring Outside the Lines: I keep my body moving!

We tend to make excuses why we can't exercise. "I'm too busy," is a common one. However, without movement it is easier to feel lethargic, depressed, and impatient. What kind of workout activities and body movement do you enjoy?

Now write out your plan on how you are going to get your body moving again! Or, if you already do, what new movement exercises do you want to try out? Make a Date Night for yourself to "get off the couch!"

Be the Connoisseur of Your Own Soul

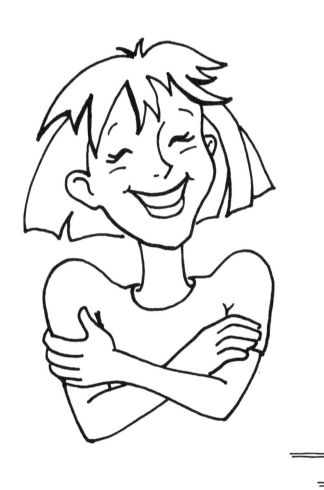

Be the Connoisseur
of Your Own Soul

Years ago I recall watching a movie with a friend during medical school. While I don't recall the title of the film, I do recall its meaning. It was about a woman who had been devastated by the loss of a marriage dream. She had married a man who had no real interest in her, and who was very neglectful of her needs and beauty. She went on a trip and ended up meeting a man who was the opposite; he did see her beauty, and over time, she fell in love with him, calling him the "connoisseur of her soul." At the time I thought that movie was so magical, and I remember my friend telling me that I needed to wait for a man like that to be in my life.

Don't get me wrong, people are important—we can't live isolated and without our relationships—but I fail to understand why we can't be our own connoisseur of our own souls. I don't know anyone who knows me as good as I know me, and I don't know anyone who could possibly know what is in my heart as well as I do or could other than the Creator.

Coloring Outside the Lines: I am perfect for me!

Don't make the mistake of relying on others for your sense of worth; you need to derive that from yourself. If you rely on someone else and they pass away, what would you do? If you are not relying on yourself for your sense of worth or value, and if you are not cultivating and enriching yourself all the time, you will drown in that loss or other family responsibilities. The best thing you can do for yourself and those around you is cultivate your best self, every day, in every way. Keep your heart at peace, go with the flow of life, work hard to accomplish your dreams, and stay rested. If you do these things, you will become your own "soul connoisseur" and you will be amazing.

I am perfect for me!

Printed in the USA
CPSIA information can be obtained
at www.ICGtesting.com
LVHW080245070324
773191LV00004BA/115